CARNIVORE

DIET COOKBOOK FOR MEN

50 Tasty, High-Protein Meat-Based Recipes that Support Muscle Growth, Testosterone Levels, and Overall Male Health

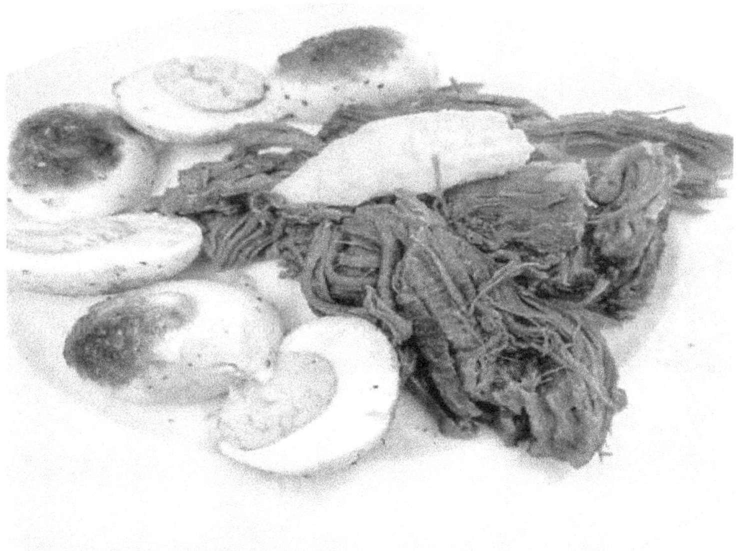

DR. COLE HULL

COPYRIGHT

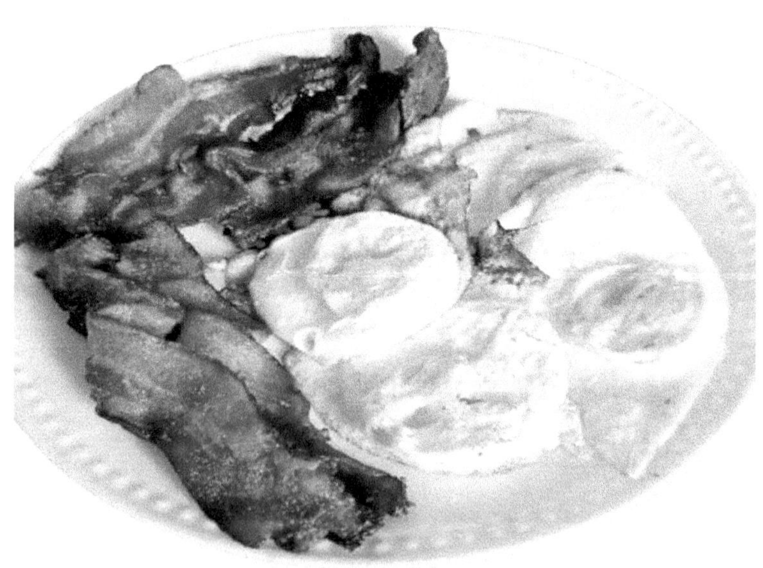

COPYRIGHT

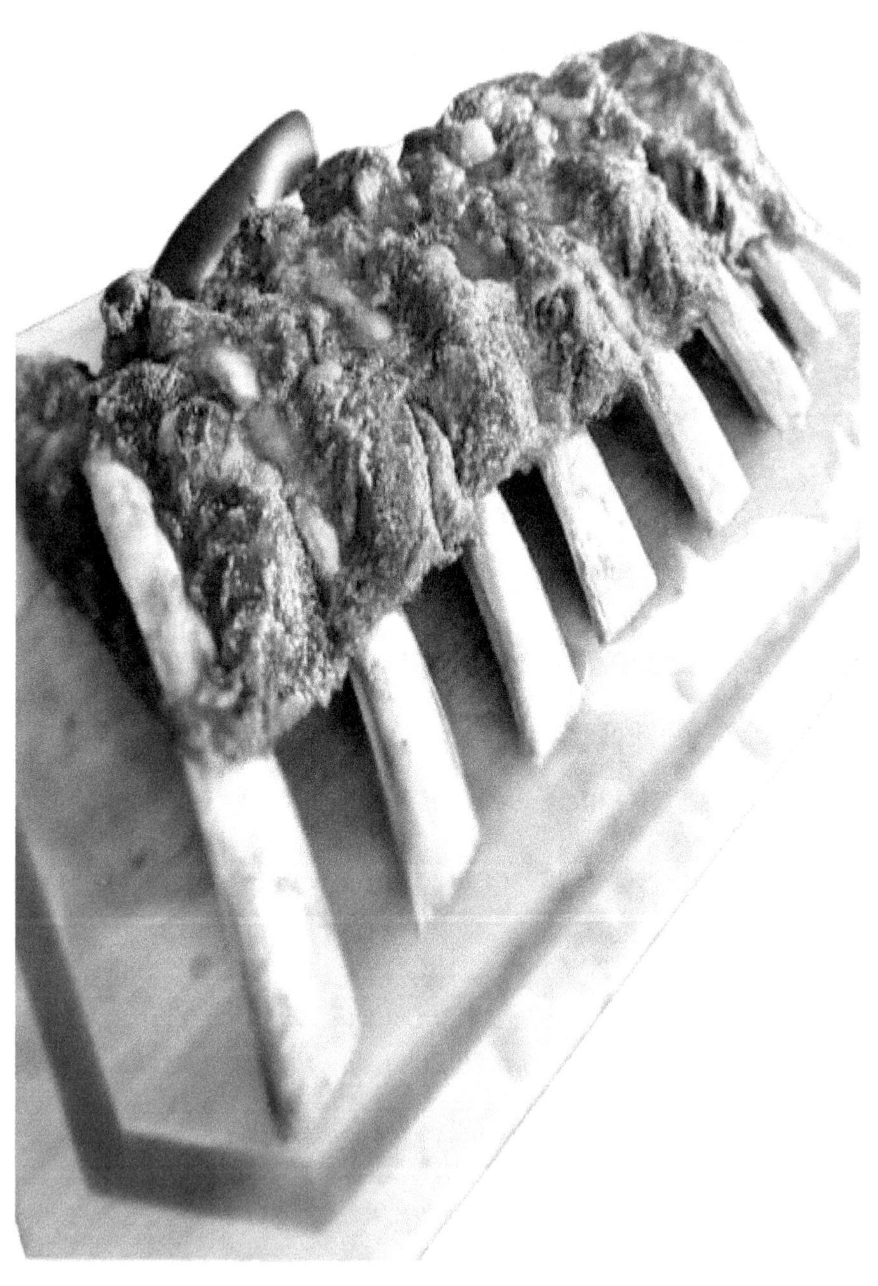

1. INTRODUCTION

Welcome, gentlemen, to a culinary adventure that strips eating back to its most primal form. This is not just another diet; it is a return to the roots of manhood, a tribute to our hunter-gatherer ancestors, and a testament to the beauty of simplicity in food. The Carnivore Diet emphasizes the consumption of animal-based foods in their purest form. It not only helps with physical transformation but also encourages a deeper understanding of the strong link between the food we eat and our inherent masculine vitality.

In this valuable cookbook, we explore the art and science of preparing and enjoying a variety of meats, fish, and animal products. Our focus is on providing nourishment for both the body and the soul. Whether you're a seasoned carnivore aficionado or a curious newcomer, this collection aims to inspire, educate, and satisfy. It features recipes that cater specifically to the nutritional and physiological needs of men.

Farewell to the era of aimless eating and meals lacking in nutritional value. Presented in this cookbook is a carefully crafted 14-day meal plan that emphasizes top-notch proteins, essential fats, and vital nutrients to promote muscle growth, testosterone levels, and overall male health. With a focus on the carnivore ethos, each recipe in this cookbook celebrates simple ingredients, minimal preparation, and maximum flavor. From the seared perfection of a ribeye steak to the delicate textures of salmon sashimi and the robust flavors of lamb burgers, you'll find a variety of dishes to satisfy your taste buds.

This cookbook serves as a manual for a lifestyle that promotes vitality, wellness, and the pleasure of indulging in meals that are both delectable and nutritious. This book celebrates the lasting influence of meat in men's diets and encourages readers to discover the significant effects of a carnivorous eating style on their physical well-being, mental focus, and emotional strength.

So, get ready to fire up your grills, sharpen those knives, and get ready for a culinary journey that pays tribute to the power and simplicity of our ancestral nourishment. Welcome to the Ultimate Carnivore Diet Cookbook for Men—where every meal is a chance to nourish your body and embrace the primal pleasure of savoring meat.

2. DELICIOUS & NUTRITIOUS ANIMAL-BASED DIET RECIPES FOR MEN

1. Seared Ribeye Steak

Prep Time: 5 minutes

Cook Time: 6-8 minutes

Ingredients:

- 1 ribeye steak (approx. 1 inch thick or about 225 grams)
- Salt (to taste, optional)

Nutritional Information (approximate):

- Calories: 640 kcal
- Protcin: 69g
- Fat: 40g
- Carbs: 0g

Preparation:

1. Let the steak reach room temperature for about 30 minutes before cooking.

2. Preheat a skillet over high heat until very hot.

3. Season the steak with salt on both sides if desired.

4. Place the steak in the skillet and cook for 3-4 minutes on each side for medium-rare, or longer for desired doneness.

5. Rest the steak for at least 5 minutes before slicing.

Health Benefit:

Rich in protein and creatine, supporting muscle mass and strength, crucial for men's physical health and testosterone levels.

2. Bacon-Wrapped Chicken Thighs

Prep Time: 10 minutes

Cook Time: 25-30 minutes

Ingredients:

- 4 chicken thighs (boneless, skinless, approximately 600 grams total)

- 8 slices of bacon

Nutritional Information (approximate for one serving):

- Calories: 450 kcal

- Protein: 35g

- Fat: 34g

- Carbs: 0g

Preparation:

1. Preheat your oven to 400°F (200°C).

2. Wrap each chicken thigh with 2 slices of bacon, securing the bacon with toothpicks if necessary.

3. Place the wrapped thighs on a baking sheet lined with parchment paper.

4. Bake in the preheated oven for 25-30 minutes, or until the bacon is crispy and the chicken is fully cooked.

5. Let the chicken rest for a few minutes before serving.

Health Benefit:

The combination of chicken and bacon provides a good balance of protein and fats, essential for testosterone production and maintaining lean muscle mass in men.

3. Crispy Pork Belly Slices

Prep Time: 5 minutes (plus time to chill if applying salt overnight)
Cook Time: 2-3 hours

Ingredients:

- 500 grams of pork belly, skin scored
- Salt (to taste, optional)

Nutritional Information (approximate for one serving):

   - Calories: 580 kcal

   - Protein: 14g

   - Fat: 58g

   - Carbs: 0g

Preparation:

   1. Optionally, rub the pork belly skin with salt and let it sit in the fridge overnight to dry out the skin.

   2. Preheat your oven to 350°F (175°C).

   3. Place the pork belly on a rack in a roasting pan, skin-side up.

   4. Roast for 2-3 hours, or until the skin is crispy and the fat has rendered.

   5. Increase the oven temperature to 450°F (230°C) for the last 15-20 minutes to crisp up the skin further.

   6. Let the pork belly cool slightly before cutting into slices and serving.

Health Benefit:

Pork belly is a high-fat food, providing energy and essential fatty acids that support testosterone synthesis, vital for men's hormonal health.

4. Smooth Beef Liver Pâté

Prep Time: 10 minutes
Cook Time: 5 minutes

Ingredients:
  - 500 grams beef liver, cleaned and trimmed
  - 100 grams butter

Nutritional Information(approximate for one serving):
  - Calories: 200 kcal
  - Protein: 27g
  - Fat: 8g
  - Carbs: 0g

Preparation:
  1. In a skillet, melt half the butter over medium heat.
  2. Add the liver and cook until browned on the outside but still slightly pink in the middle.
  3. Transfer the liver and remaining butter to a blender and blend until smooth.
  4. Optionally, season with salt to taste and blend again.
  5. Refrigerate until firm and serve chilled.

Health Benefit:

Beef liver is packed with vitamins and minerals, especially vitamin B12 and iron, which are crucial for energy metabolism and preventing anemia, supporting overall vitality in men.

5. Egg and Ham Muffins

Prep Time: 5 minutes
Cook Time: 20 minutes
Ingredients:

  - 6 eggs

  - 6 slices of ham

Nutritional Information (approximate for one muffin):

  - Calories: 150 kcal

  - Protein: 14g

  - Fat: 10g

  - Carbs: 1g

Preparation:

  1. Preheat the oven to 350°F (175°C).

  2. Line each muffin tin with a slice of ham.

  3. Crack an egg into each ham-lined muffin cup.

  4. Bake for 15-20 minutes, or until the eggs are set.

  5. Remove from the oven and let cool for a few minutes before serving.

Health Benefit:

Eggs are an excellent source of choline, which is essential for brain health, and the combination with ham provides a satisfying balance of protein and fat, supporting muscle maintenance and overall health.

6. Chilled Salmon Sashimi

Prep Time: 10 minutes
Cook Time: 0 minutes
Ingredients:

- 200 grams fresh, high-quality salmon fillet

Nutritional Information (approximate for the whole fillet):

- Calories: 400 kcal
- Protein: 40g
- Fat: 24g
- Carbs: 0g

Preparation:

1. Ensure the salmon is very fresh and of sashimi grade.
2. Slice the salmon fillet thinly against the grain.
3. Serve immediately, chilled.

Health Benefit:

Salmon is rich in omega-3 fatty acids, which are beneficial for heart health and reducing inflammation, crucial for men as they age.

7. Grilled Lamb Chops

Prep Time: 5 minutes
Cook Time: 10 minutes
Ingredients:

  - 4 lamb chops (approximately 200 grams each)

Nutritional Information (approximate for one chop):
  - Calories: 330 kcal
  - Protein: 25g
  - Fat: 25g
  - Carbs: 0g

Preparation:
  1. Preheat your grill to high heat.
  2. Place lamb chops on the grill and cook for 3-5 minutes per side, depending on desired doneness.
  3. Let the chops rest for a few minutes before serving.

Health Benefit:

Lamb is a great source of high-quality protein and essential nutrients like zinc, supporting muscle growth and testosterone levels in men.

8. Classic Beef Tartare

Prep Time: 15 minutes
Cook Time: 0 minutes
Ingredients:

- 200 grams high-quality beef tenderloin, finely chopped
- 1 egg yolk

Nutritional Information (approximate for the entire dish):

- Calories: 500 kcal
- Protein: 40g
- Fat: 35g
- Carbs: 0g

Preparation:

1. Ensure the beef is very fresh and of high quality.
2. Mix the finely chopped beef with the egg yolk gently.
3. Shape the mixture into a patty and serve immediately.

Health Benefit:

Beef tenderloin is lean and rich in iron and vitamin B12, essential for energy and maintaining healthy blood cells, crucial for men's health.

9. Carnivore Scotch Eggs

Prep Time: 10 minutes

Cook Time: 30 minutes

Ingredients:

- 6 eggs, hard-boiled
- 300 grams ground sausage meat

Nutritional Information (approximate for one scotch egg):

- Calories: 300 kcal
- Protein: 20g
- Fat: 22g
- Carbs: 1g

Preparation:

1. Preheat your oven to 350°F (175°C).
2. Peel the hard-boiled eggs.
3. Flatten a portion of the sausage meat and wrap it around each egg, ensuring it's fully covered.

4. Place the sausage-wrapped eggs on a baking sheet and bake for 20-25 minutes until the meat is cooked through.

5. Let them cool slightly before serving.

Health Benefit:

Eggs and sausage provide a high-quality protein source, essential for muscle repair and growth, beneficial for men engaged in regular physical activity.

10. Butter-Basted Scallops

Prep Time: 5 minutes
Cook Time: 6 minutes
Ingredients:

- 12 sea scallops
- 50 grams butter

Nutritional Information (approximate for 3 scallops):

- Calories: 200 kcal
- Protein: 14g
- Fat: 15g
- Carbs: 0g

Preparation:

1. Pat the scallops dry with a paper towel.

2. Heat a skillet over medium-high heat and add the butter.

3. Once the butter is melted and foamy, add the scallops, making sure not to overcrowd the pan.

4. Cook for about 2-3 minutes on one side, until a golden crust forms, then flip and baste with the melted butter for another 2-3 minutes.

5. Serve immediately.

Health Benefit:

Scallops are an excellent source of protein and omega-3 fatty acids, promoting heart health and reducing inflammation, important for men's cardiovascular health.

11. Duck Breast with Crispy Skin

Prep Time: 5 minutes

Cook Time: 15 minutes

Ingredients:

- 2 duck breasts (approximately 200 grams each)

Nutritional Information (approximate for one breast):

- Calories: 400 kcal

- Protein: 30g

- Fat: 30g

- Carbs: 0g

Preparation:

1. Score the skin of the duck breasts in a diamond pattern.

2. Place them skin side down in a cold skillet.

3. Turn the heat to medium and cook for 6-8 minutes until the skin is crispy.

4. Flip the breasts over and cook for another 5-7 minutes.

5. Let them rest for 5 minutes before slicing.

Health Benefit:

Duck is a rich source of protein and B vitamins, essential for energy metabolism and muscle maintenance, beneficial for men's health.

12. Pork Rind Nachos

Prep Time: 5 minutes

Cook Time: 10 minutes

Ingredients:

- 100 grams pork rinds

- 200 grams shredded cheese (e.g., cheddar or mozzarella)

- 200 grams cooked chicken breast, shredded

Nutritional Information (approximate for a serving):

  - Calories: 600 kcal

  - Protein: 60g

  - Fat: 40g

  - Carbs: 1g

Preparation:

  1. Preheat your oven to 350°F (175°C).

  2. Spread pork rinds on a baking sheet.

  3. Top with shredded cheese and chicken.

  4. Bake until the cheese is melted and bubbly, about 8-10 minutes.

  5. Serve immediately.

Health Benefit:

This dish provides a high protein content with minimal carbs, supporting muscle synthesis and maintenance, crucial for men's physical health.

13. Fresh Oysters

Prep Time: 10 minutes

Cook Time: 0 minutes

Ingredients:

- 12 fresh oysters

- Nutritional Information (approximate for 3 oysters):

  - Calories: 50 kcal

  - Protein: 6g

  - Fat: 2g

  - Carbs: 3g

Preparation:

1. Scrub the oyster shells clean under cold water.

2. Use an oyster knife to carefully shuck the oysters, keeping the liquor inside.

3. Serve on a bed of ice.

Health Benefit:

Oysters are a powerhouse of zinc, crucial for testosterone production and reproductive health in men.

14. Chicken Liver Fried in Duck Fat

Prep Time: 5 minutes

Cook Time: 8 minutes

Ingredients:

  - 300 grams chicken livers, cleaned

  - 50 grams duck fat

Nutritional Information (approximate for a serving):

  - Calories: 360 kcal

  - Protein: 45g

  - Fat: 18g

  - Carbs: 0g

Preparation:

  1. Heat the duck fat in a skillet over medium heat.

  2. Add the chicken livers and cook for 3-4 minutes on each side until browned but still slightly pink in the middle.

  3. Serve immediately.

Health Benefit:

Chicken liver is rich in iron and vitamins, supporting energy levels and cognitive function, which is beneficial for men's overall well-being.

15. Smoked Whole Trout

Prep Time: 10 minutes (plus time for smoking)

Cook Time: 1-2 hours (depending on smoker)

Ingredients:

- 2 whole trout, cleaned

Nutritional Information (approximate for one trout):

- Calories: 380 kcal

- Protein: 56g

- Fat: 18g

- Carbs: 0g

Preparation:

1. Preheat your smoker to 225°F (107°C).

2. Place the whole trout in the smoker.

3. Smoke for 1-2 hours, or until the fish is cooked through and flakes easily.

4. Serve immediately.

Health Benefit:

Trout is high in omega-3 fatty acids, beneficial for heart health and reducing inflammation, important for maintaining men's cardiovascular health.

16. Quail Grilled to Perfection

Prep Time: 5 minutes

Cook Time: 10-12 minutes

Ingredients:

- 4 quails, cleaned and prepped for grilling

Nutritional Information (approximate for one quail):

- Calories: 123 kcal

- Protein: 21g

- Fat: 4g

- Carbs: 0g

Preparation:

1. Preheat the grill to medium-high heat.

2. Place quails on the grill and cook for 5-6 minutes per side, until the skin is crispy and the meat is cooked through.

3. Let them rest for a few minutes before serving.

Health Benefit:

Quail provides a lean source of protein, which is essential for muscle repair and building, crucial for men's physical health and fitness.

17. Nutritious Beef Bone Broth

Prep Time: 10 minutes (plus simmering time)

Cook Time: 24-48 hours

Ingredients:

- 2 kg beef bones (preferably a mix of marrow bones and bones with a bit of meat)

- Water to cover

Nutritional Information (approximate for 1 cup):

- Calories: 40 kcal

- Protein: 6g

- Fat: 1g

- Carbs: 0g

Preparation:

1. Place beef bones in a large stockpot and cover with water.

2. Bring to a boil, then reduce heat and simmer for 24-48 hours, skimming off any foam that forms.

3. Strain the broth, cool, and store in the refrigerator or freezer.

Health Benefit:

Bone broth is rich in collagen and minerals, supporting joint health and digestion, which is beneficial for men's long-term well-being and athletic performance.

18. Bacon and Egg Breakfast Cups

Prep Time: 5 minutes

Cook Time: 15-20 minutes

Ingredients:

- 12 slices of bacon

- 12 eggs

Nutritional Information (approximate for one cup):

- Calories: 150 kcal

- Protein: 12g

- Fat: 11g

- Carbs: 1g

Preparation:

1. Preheat the oven to 375°F (190°C).

2. Line each muffin tin with a slice of bacon, forming a ring.

3. Crack an egg into each bacon-lined cup.

4. Bake for 15-20 minutes, or until the egg whites are set and the yolks are cooked to your liking.

5. Allow to cool slightly before removing from the tin and serving.

Health Benefit:

A great source of protein and healthy fats, this meal supports testosterone levels and muscle maintenance, essential for men's health.

19. Homemade Venison Jerky

Prep Time: 15 minutes (plus marinating time)
Cook Time: 3-8 hours (depending on dehydrator)
Ingredients:

- 1 kg venison, sliced thinly against the grain

Nutritional Information (approximate for 100g):

- Calories: 250 kcal

- Protein: 33g

- Fat: 3g

- Carbs: 0g

Preparation:

1. Place venison slices in a single layer in a dehydrator.

2. Dehydrate at 160°F (70°C) for 3-8 hours, or until the jerky is dry and leathery.

3. Store in an airtight container.

Health Benefit:

Venison jerky is a lean, high-protein snack that supports muscle building and repair, ideal for men's fitness and recovery.

20. Blue Cheese Pork Chops

Prep Time: 5 minutes

Cook Time: 12-15 minutes

Ingredients:

- 4 pork chops (approximately 200 grams each)
- 100 grams blue cheese, crumbled

Nutritional Information (approximate for one chop with cheese):

- Calories: 350 kcal
- Protein: 35g
- Fat: 22g
- Carbs: 1g

Preparation:

1. Preheat your grill or skillet over medium-high heat.

2. Grill the pork chops for 5-7 minutes on each side, or until they reach the desired level of doneness.

3. In the last few minutes of cooking, top each chop with blue cheese, allowing it to melt slightly.

4. Serve hot, with the melted blue cheese on top.

Health Benefit:

This dish combines high-quality protein from pork with the benefits of blue cheese, which includes calcium and beneficial fats, supporting bone health and providing a satisfying, nutrient-dense meal for men.

21. Steamed Crab Legs with Melted Butter

Prep Time: 5 minutes
Cook Time: 10 minutes
Ingredients:

- 1 kg crab legs, pre-cooked and frozen
- 100 grams butter

Nutritional Information (approximate for 100g serving):

- Calories: 130 kcal
- Protein: 26g
- Fat: 2g
- Carbs: 0g

Preparation:

1. Thaw the crab legs if frozen.

2. Bring a large pot of water to a boil and place a steamer basket over it.

3. Add the crab legs to the basket, cover, and steam for about 10 minutes until heated through.

4. Melt the butter in a separate pot or microwave.

5. Serve the crab legs with melted butter for dipping.

Health Benefit:

Crab legs are an excellent source of high-quality protein and omega-3 fatty acids, supporting heart health and muscle maintenance, crucial for men's overall well-being.

22. Raw Steak Tartare with Egg Yolk

Prep Time: 15 minutes

Cook Time: 0 minutes

Ingredients:

- 200 grams high-quality beef tenderloin, finely chopped
- 1 egg yolk

Nutritional Information (approximate for the entire dish):

- Calories: 500 kcal
- Protein: 40g

- Fat: 35g

- Carbs: 0g

Preparation:

1. Ensure the beef is very fresh and of high quality.

2. Mix the finely chopped beef with the egg yolk gently.

3. Shape the mixture into a patty and serve immediately.

Health Benefit:

Steak tartare provides a rich source of heme iron and protein, essential for oxygen transport and muscle growth, particularly beneficial for men's physical health and energy levels.

23. Grilled Bison Burgers

Prep Time: 10 minutes

Cook Time: 10 minutes

Ingredients:

- 500 grams ground bison

Nutritional Information (approximate for one burger):

- Calories: 280 kcal

- Protein: 40g

- Fat: 12g

- Carbs: 0g

Preparation:

1. Preheat the grill to high heat.

2. Form the ground bison into 4 equal-sized patties.

3. Grill the patties for about 5 minutes per side, or to desired doneness.

4. Serve immediately.

Health Benefit:

Bison meat is leaner than beef and provides a good source of protein and iron, supporting muscle maintenance and cardiovascular health, which is key for men's health.

24. Crispy Chicken Wings

Prep Time: 5 minutes

Cook Time: 45 minutes

Ingredients:

- 1 kg chicken wings

Nutritional Information (approximate for 100g serving):

- Calories: 290 kcal

- Protein: 24g

- Fat: 20g

- Carbs: 0g

Preparation:

1. Preheat the oven to 400°F (200°C).

2. Place the chicken wings on a baking sheet in a single layer.

3. Bake for 45 minutes, or until the skin is crispy and the wings are fully cooked.

4. Serve immediately.

Health Benefit:

Chicken wings are a great source of protein and fats, which are essential for testosterone production and muscle repair, important for men's health and fitness.

25. Roasted Beef Bone Marrow

Prep Time: 5 minutes

Cook Time: 20 minutes

Ingredients:

- 4 beef marrow bones, cut lengthwise

Nutritional Information (approximate for one serving):

- Calories: 110 kcal

- Protein: 7g

- Fat: 9g

- Carbs: 0g

Preparation:

1. Preheat the oven to 450°F (230°C).

2. Place the marrow bones on a baking sheet, marrow side up.

3. Roast in the preheated oven for about 20 minutes, or until the marrow is soft and slightly bubbly.

4. Serve immediately, scooping out the marrow with a small spoon.

Health Benefit:

Bone marrow is rich in fatty acids, vitamins, and minerals, supporting immune health and providing essential nutrients for bone health and cellular repair, beneficial for men's overall vitality.

26. Pan-Fried Fish Roe

Prep Time: 5 minutes

Cook Time: 4 minutes

Ingredients:

- 200 grams fish roe (such as salmon or cod roe)

Nutritional Information (approximate for 100g serving):

- Calories: 143 kcal

- Protein: 29g

- Fat: 6g

- Carbs: 0g

Preparation:

1. Gently rinse the fish roe under cold water and pat dry.

2. Heat a non-stick skillet over medium heat.

3. Carefully add the roe to the skillet and fry for 2 minutes on each side until slightly crispy on the outside.

4. Serve immediately.

Health Benefit:

Fish roe is an excellent source of omega-3 fatty acids and vitamin D, crucial for cardiovascular health and testosterone production, which are important for men's health.

27. Oven-Roasted Rack of Lamb

Prep Time: 5 minutes

Cook Time: 25 minutes

Ingredients:

- 1 rack of lamb (approx. 500 grams)

Nutritional Information (approximate for 100g serving):

- Calories: 258 kcal

- Protein: 25g

- Fat: 17g

- Carbs: 0g

Preparation:

1. Preheat the oven to 400°F (200°C).

2. Place the rack of lamb on a roasting tray.

3. Roast in the preheated oven for 20-25 minutes for medium-rare.

4. Let it rest for 10 minutes before carving between the ribs and serving.

Health Benefit:

Lamb is a rich source of high-quality protein and zinc, essential for muscle growth, repair, and overall immune function, which are particularly important for men's health.

28. Sautéed Shrimp in Butter

Prep Time: 5 minutes

Cook Time: 6 minutes

Ingredients:

- 400 grams shrimp, peeled and deveined
- 50 grams butter

Nutritional Information (approximate for 100g serving):

- Calories: 240 kcal
- Protein: 24g

- Fat: 15g

- Carbs: 1g

Preparation:

1. Melt the butter in a large skillet over medium heat.

2. Add the shrimp and cook for 2-3 minutes per side until they turn pink and opaque.

3. Serve immediately.

Health Benefit:

Shrimp are low in calories yet high in protein and selenium, supporting muscle health and antioxidant defense, which is crucial for men's health and fitness.

29. Cheese-Stuffed Carnivore Omelet

Prep Time: 5 minutes

Cook Time: 5 minutes

Ingredients:

- 3 eggs

- 100 grams cheese of your choice, shredded

Nutritional Information (approximate for the entire omelet):

- Calories: 470 kcal

- Protein: 33g

- Fat: 36g

- Carbs: 3g

Preparation:

1. Beat the eggs in a bowl and pour into a heated non-stick skillet over medium heat.

2. Once the eggs begin to set, sprinkle cheese on one half.

3. Fold the omelet over the cheese and cook until the cheese is melted.

4. Serve immediately.

Health Benefit:

This high-protein, high-fat meal is ideal for muscle maintenance and provides sustained energy, crucial for men's physical activity and metabolic health.

30. Grilled Whole Sardines

Prep Time: 5 minutes

Cook Time: 6 minutes

Ingredients:

- 8 whole sardines, cleaned

Nutritional Information (approximate for 2 sardines):

- Calories: 150 kcal

- Protein: 17g

- Fat: 9g

- Carbs: 0g

Preparation:

1. Preheat the grill to medium-high heat.

2. Grill the sardines for 2-3 minutes on each side until the skin is crispy and the fish is cooked through.

3. Serve immediately.

Health Benefit:

Sardines are an excellent source of omega-3 fatty acids, protein, and calcium, supporting heart health, bone density, and muscle function, which are essential for men's overall well-being.

31. Sausage and Egg Skillet

Prep Time: 5 minutes

Cook Time: 10 minutes

Ingredients:

- 4 large eggs

- 200 grams sausage, sliced

Nutritional Information (approximate for one serving):

- Calories: 320 kcal

- Protein: 22g

- Fat: 24g

- Carbs: 1g

Preparation:

1. Heat a skillet over medium heat and cook the sausage slices until browned and cooked through.

2. Crack the eggs directly into the skillet with the sausage and cook to your desired level of doneness.

3. Serve hot straight from the skillet.

Health Benefit:

This hearty meal provides a high protein and fat content, ideal for supporting testosterone levels and muscle synthesis, important for men's health.

32. Caviar-Topped Deviled Eggs

Prep Time: 10 minutes

Cook Time: 10 minutes

Ingredients:

- 6 large eggs, hard-boiled and halved
- 30 grams caviar

Nutritional Information (approximate for one egg half):

- Calories: 60 kcal
- Protein: 6g
- Fat: 4g
- Carbs: 0g

Preparation:

1. Remove the yolks from the hard-boiled eggs and set the whites aside.

2. Mash the yolks with a fork and spoon them back into the egg whites.

3. Top each egg half with a small spoonful of caviar.

4. Serve chilled.

Health Benefit:

Caviar is a luxurious source of omega-3 fatty acids and vitamin B12, crucial for cardiovascular health and energy metabolism, beneficial for men's health.

33. Seared Ribeye Cap Steak

Prep Time: 5 minutes

Cook Time: 8 minutes

Ingredients:

- 2 ribeye cap steaks (approximately 200 grams each)

Nutritional Information (approximate for one steak):

- Calories: 500 kcal

- Protein: 40g

- Fat: 38g

- Carbs: 0g

Preparation:

1. Heat a skillet over high heat until very hot.

2. Sear the steaks for 3-4 minutes on each side for medium-rare, or to your desired level of doneness.

3. Let the steaks rest for a few minutes before serving.

Health Benefit:

The ribeye cap is rich in protein and healthy fats, including omega-3s, which are essential for muscle maintenance and hormonal health in men.

34. Slow-Cooked Pulled Pork

Prep Time: 10 minutes
Cook Time: 8 hours
Ingredients:
  - 1 kg pork shoulder

Nutritional Information (approximate for 100g serving):
  - Calories: 276 kcal
  - Protein: 30g
  - Fat: 16g
  - Carbs: 0g

Preparation:
  1. Place the pork shoulder in a slow cooker.
  2. Cook on low for 8 hours or until the meat is tender and shreds easily.
  3. Shred the pork with two forks and serve.

Health Benefit:

Pulled pork is an excellent source of high-quality protein, supporting tissue repair and muscle growth, which is crucial for men's physical health and recovery.

35. Tender Smoked Chicken

Prep Time: 10 minutes (plus brining time if desired)

Cook Time: 3-4 hours

Ingredients:

- 1 whole chicken (approximately 1.5 kg)

Nutritional Information (approximate for 100g serving):

- Calories: 215 kcal

- Protein: 18g

- Fat: 15g

- Carbs: 0g

Preparation:

1. Preheat your smoker to 225°F (107°C).

2. Place the whole chicken in the smoker.

3. Smoke for 3-4 hours, or until the internal temperature reaches 165°F (74°C).

4. Let the chicken rest for 10 minutes before carving and serving.

Health Benefit:

Smoked chicken provides a lean source of protein and essential nutrients, aiding in muscle repair and maintenance, and supporting immune function, key for men's health.

36. Grilled Swordfish Steaks

Prep Time: 5 minutes
Cook Time: 10 minutes
Ingredients:

- 2 swordfish steaks (approximately 200 grams each)

Nutritional Information (approximate for one steak):

- Calories: 235 kcal
- Protein: 33g
- Fat: 10g
- Carbs: 0g

Preparation:

1. Preheat your grill to medium-high heat.

2. Grill the swordfish steaks for 4-5 minutes on each side, or until the fish flakes easily with a fork.

3. Serve immediately.

Health Benefit:

Swordfish is a hearty, meaty fish that's high in protein and omega-3 fatty acids, beneficial for heart health and reducing inflammation, important for men's health.

37. Duck Legs Confit

Prep Time: 10 minutes (plus overnight for seasoning if desired)
Cook Time: 4 hours
Ingredients:

  - 4 duck legs

  - Duck fat, enough to cover the legs

Nutritional Information (approximate for one leg):

  - Calories: 320 kcal

  - Protein: 27g

  - Fat: 24g

  - Carbs: 0g

Preparation:

  1. Optional: Season the duck legs with salt and let them rest in the fridge overnight.

  2. Preheat your oven to 275°F (135°C).

3. Rinse the salt off the duck legs (if seasoned overnight) and pat them dry.

4. Place the legs in a baking dish and cover them completely with melted duck fat.

5. Cook in the oven for 3-4 hours or until the meat is very tender.

6. Serve the duck legs with the skin crisped up under a broiler if desired.

Health Benefit:

Duck confit is rich in monounsaturated fats and provides a good source of protein, supporting muscle health and providing sustained energy, key for active men.

38. Grilled Tuna Steaks

Prep Time: 5 minutes

Cook Time: 6 minutes

Ingredients:

- 2 tuna steaks (approximately 200 grams each)

Nutritional Information (approximate for one steak):

- Calories: 220 kcal

- Protein: 40g

- Fat: 5g

- Carbs: 0g

Preparation:

1. Preheat your grill to high heat.

2. Grill the tuna steaks for 2-3 minutes on each side, keeping the center pink for medium-rare.

3. Serve immediately.

Health Benefit:

Tuna is an excellent source of high-quality protein and omega-3 fatty acids, which support cardiovascular health and muscle maintenance, crucial for men's fitness and well-being.

39. Roasted Whole Goose

Prep Time: 15 minutes

Cook Time: 3 hours

Ingredients:

- 1 whole goose (approximately 4-5 kg)

Nutritional Information(approximate for 100g serving):

- Calories: 340 kcal

- Protein: 29g

- Fat: 24g

- Carbs: 0g

Preparation:

1. Preheat your oven to 350°F (175°C).

2. Prick the goose skin all over with a fork to help render the fat.

3. Roast in the oven for about 3 hours, or until the internal temperature reaches 165°F (74°C) and the skin is crisp.

4. Let the goose rest for 20 minutes before carving and serving.

Health Benefit:

Goose provides a rich source of iron and B vitamins, essential for energy production and maintaining healthy blood cells, supporting men's active lifestyles.

40. Bacon-Wrapped Scallops

Prep Time: 10 minutes

Cook Time: 15 minutes

Ingredients:

- 12 large scallops
- 12 slices of bacon

Nutritional Information (approximate for 3 wrapped scallops):

- Calories: 315 kcal
- Protein: 18g
- Fat: 24g
- Carbs: 1g

Preparation:

1. Preheat your oven to 400°F (200°C).

2. Wrap each scallop with a slice of bacon and secure with a toothpick.

3. Bake in the preheated oven for 15 minutes, or until the bacon is crispy and the scallops are opaque.

4. Serve immediately.

Health Benefit:

Scallops wrapped in bacon offer a high-protein, nutrient-rich snack or appetizer, with the omega-3 fatty acids from scallops and the protein from bacon supporting muscle growth and cardiovascular health.

41. Lamb Burgers

Prep Time: 10 minutes

Cook Time: 10 minutes

Ingredients:

- 500 grams ground lamb

Nutritional Information (approximate for one burger):

- Calories: 330 kcal

- Protein: 30g

- Fat: 22g

- Carbs: 0g

Preparation:

1. Preheat your grill or skillet to medium-high heat.

2. Form the ground lamb into 4 equal-sized patties.

3. Grill or cook the patties for about 5 minutes on each side, or until they reach your desired level of doneness.

4. Serve immediately.

Health Benefit:

Lamb is rich in high-quality protein and essential nutrients like iron and zinc, which are crucial for muscle growth, repair, and overall men's health.

42. Fried Chicken Skins

Prep Time: 5 minutes

Cook Time: 10 minutes

Ingredients:

- Chicken skins from 6 thighs or breasts

Nutritional Information (approximate for a serving):

- Calories: 150 kcal

- Protein: 15g

- Fat: 10g

- Carbs: 0g

Preparation:

1. Heat a skillet over medium heat.

2. Add the chicken skins, fat side down, and cook until the fat renders and the skins become crispy, about 5 minutes per side.

3. Serve immediately.

Health Benefit:

Chicken skins provide a crunchy, satisfying source of fats and protein, supporting satiety and energy levels, which are important for maintaining men's health.

43. Bacon and Egg Salad

Prep Time: 10 minutes

Cook Time: 10 minutes

Ingredients:

- 6 eggs, hard-boiled and chopped

- 200 grams bacon, cooked and crumbled

Nutritional Information (approximate for one serving):

- Calories: 320 kcal

- Protein: 25g

- Fat: 24g

- Carbs: 1g

Preparation:

1. Mix the chopped eggs and crumbled bacon in a bowl.

2. Serve as is or over a bed of lettuce if desired for a crunch (keeping in mind lettuce is not carnivore).

3. Serve immediately or chilled.

Health Benefit:

This high-protein salad supports muscle repair and growth. The fats from the eggs and bacon contribute to hormone regulation, including testosterone, which is vital for men's health.

44. Pork Rind-Crusted Cod

Prep Time: 10 minutes

Cook Time: 15 minutes

Ingredients:

- 4 cod fillets (approximately 150 grams each)

- 100 grams crushed pork rinds

Nutritional Information (approximate for one fillet):

- Calories: 220 kcal

- Protein: 40g

- Fat: 5g

- Carbs: 0g

Preparation:

1. Preheat your oven to 400°F (200°C).

2. Coat each cod fillet in crushed pork rinds and place on a baking sheet.

3. Bake for 15 minutes, or until the fish flakes easily with a fork.

4. Serve immediately.

Health Benefit:

Cod is a lean source of protein, supporting muscle maintenance and growth. The pork rind crust adds healthy fats for energy and satiety, important for men's metabolic health.

45. Beef Cheek Barbacoa

Prep Time: 15 minutes
Cook Time: 8 hours
Ingredients:

- 1 kg beef cheeks, trimmed

Nutritional Information (approximate for 100g serving):

- Calories: 250 kcal

- Protein: 32g

- Fat: 12g

- Carbs: 0g

Preparation:

1. Place beef cheeks in a slow cooker.

2. Cook on low for 8 hours or until the meat is tender and easily shreds.

3. Shred the beef cheeks and serve.

Health Benefit:

Beef cheeks are rich in collagen, which supports joint health and skin elasticity. The high protein content aids in muscle recovery and growth, essential for men's fitness and overall well-being.

46. Fried Frog Legs

Prep Time: 10 minutes

Cook Time: 10 minutes

Ingredients:

- 8 frog legs

Nutritional Information (approximate for 2 frog legs):

- Calories: 150 kcal

- Protein: 30g

- Fat: 1g

- Carbs: 0g

Preparation:

1. Pat the frog legs dry with paper towels.

2. Heat a skillet over medium-high heat.

3. Cook the frog legs for 4-5 minutes on each side until they are golden brown and the meat is tender.

4. Serve immediately.

Health Benefit:

Frog legs are a lean source of protein, which is crucial for muscle repair and building. They also contain omega-3 fatty acids, beneficial for heart health and reducing inflammation, important for men's health.

47. Smoked Eel Fillets

Prep Time: 5 minutes (plus brining time if applicable)

Cook Time: 2 hours

Ingredients:

- 2 whole eels, cleaned and filleted

Nutritional Information (approximate for 1 fillet):

- Calories: 375 kcal

- Protein: 36g

- Fat: 24g

- Carbs: 0g

Preparation:

1. Preheat your smoker to 225°F (107°C).

2. Place the eel fillets in the smoker.

3. Smoke for 2 hours, or until the eel is cooked through and has a slightly crispy exterior.

4. Serve immediately.

Health Benefit:

Eel is high in omega-3 fatty acids, which are essential for cardiovascular health and cognitive function. It's also a great source of protein, supporting muscle maintenance and growth.

48. Char-Grilled Octopus

Prep Time: 15 minutes (plus precooking time)

Cook Time: 6 minutes

Ingredients:

- 1 whole octopus, cleaned and pre-cooked until tender

Nutritional Information (approximate for 100g serving):

- Calories: 164 kcal

- Protein: 30g

- Fat: 2g

- Carbs: 0g

Preparation:

1. Preheat your grill to high heat.

2. Char-grill the pre-cooked octopus for 2-3 minutes on each side until crispy and slightly charred.

3. Serve immediately.

Health Benefit:

Octopus is a low-fat, high-protein seafood that's rich in iron and B vitamins, supporting energy levels and muscle health, which are crucial for men's physical fitness and endurance.

49. Elk Meatballs

Prep Time: 20 minutes

Cook Time: 20 minutes

Ingredients:

- 500 grams ground elk meat

Nutritional Information (approximate for 4 meatballs):

- Calories: 250 kcal

- Protein: 35g

- Fat: 12g

- Carbs: 0g

Preparation:

1. Preheat your oven to 375°F (190°C).

2. Form the ground elk into meatballs and place them on a baking sheet.

3. Bake for 20 minutes, or until the meatballs are cooked through.

4. Serve immediately.

Health Benefit:

Elk meat is a lean, nutrient-dense source of protein, rich in iron and B vitamins, which helps in muscle building and maintaining energy levels, beneficial for men's health.

50. Crispy Pork Rind Pancakes

Prep Time: 5 minutes

Cook Time: 10 minutes

Ingredients:

- 100 grams crushed pork rinds

- 4 eggs, beaten

Nutritional Information (approximate for 2 pancakes):

- Calories: 300 kcal

- Protein: 28g

- Fat: 20g

- Carbs: 0g

Preparation:

1. Mix the crushed pork rinds with the beaten eggs until a batter forms.

2. Heat a non-stick skillet over medium heat.

3. Pour small amounts of the batter into the skillet, cooking for about 2-3 minutes on each side until golden brown.

4. Serve immediately.

Health Benefit:

These unique pancakes offer a high-protein, low-carb alternative, supporting muscle maintenance and satiety. The high collagen content in pork rinds also supports joint health and skin elasticity, important for men's overall well-being.

3. A FLEXIBLE 14-DAY CARNIVORE DIET MEAL PLAN FOR MEN

Day 1

- Breakfast: Bacon and Egg Breakfast Cups

- Lunch: Grilled Lamb Chops

- Dinner: Seared Ribeye Steak

Day 2

- Breakfast: Egg and Ham Muffins

- Lunch: Smoked Whole Trout

- Dinner: Classic Beef Tartare

Day 3

- Breakfast: Carnivore Scotch Eggs

- Lunch: Grilled Sardines

- Dinner: Duck Breast with Crispy Skin

Day 4

- Breakfast: Crispy Pork Belly Slices

- Lunch: Smoked Chicken

- Dinner: Pork Rind Nachos with Shredded Cheese and Chicken

Day 5

- Breakfast: Caviar-Topped Deviled Eggs

- Lunch: Bacon-Wrapped Chicken Thighs

- Dinner: Bison Burgers

Day 6

- Breakfast: Fried Fish Roe

- Lunch: Beef Liver Pâté

- Dinner: Lamb Burger

Day 7

- Breakfast: Fried Frog Legs

- Lunch: Grilled Quail

- Dinner: Beef Cheek Barbacoa

Day 8

- Breakfast: Chilled Salmon Sashimi

- Lunch: Rack of Lamb

- Dinner: Bacon-Wrapped Scallops

Day 9

- Breakfast: Crispy Chicken Wings

- Lunch: Grilled Swordfish Steaks

- Dinner: Pulled Pork

Day 10

- Breakfast: Butter-Basted Scallops

- Lunch: Char-Grilled Octopus

- Dinner: Roast Goose

Day 11

- Breakfast: Sausage and Egg Skillet

- Lunch: Beef Bone Marrow

- Dinner: Duck Legs Confit

Day 12

- Breakfast: Bacon and Egg Salad

- Lunch: Tuna Steaks with Wasabi (optional wasabi)

- Dinner: Venison Jerky as a snack, Elk Meatballs for the main meal

Day 13

- Breakfast: Pork Rind-Crusted Cod

- Lunch: Fresh Oysters

- Dinner: Smoked Eel Fillets

Day 14

- Breakfast: Crispy Pork Rind Pancakes

- Lunch: Nutritious Beef Bone Broth (can be consumed as a drink

or soup base)

- Dinner: Ribeye Cap Steak

This meal plan offers a wide range of meat, fish, and seafood options to provide a diverse array of nutrients, flavors, and textures. It aligns with the carnivore diet's focus on animal-based foods.

Don't forget, staying hydrated is crucial, so make sure to drink enough water throughout the day. Before embarking on a new diet plan, it's advisable to seek guidance from a healthcare professional if you have any dietary restrictions or health concerns.

4. CONCLUSION

As we reach the end of this cookbook, it becomes evident that it offers more than just a compilation of recipes. It serves as a guide to a lifestyle that embraces the primal essence of manhood. Every recipe, whether it's a perfectly cooked steak or butter-basted scallops, highlights the important link between our well-being, energy, and the food we eat.

Embarking on this carnivore journey is not just about adopting a diet; it's about respecting the timeless wisdom that has nourished people for generations. It's all about understanding the incredible benefits of whole, unprocessed, animal-based foods for our bodies, minds, and spirits. The recipes you've explored and the meal plans you've followed are guiding you towards a more vibrant and robust version of yourself.

This cookbook is designed to empower you with the necessary tools to not only nourish yourself, but to flourish. The nutritional principles presented in this cookbook are focused on the carnivore diet's emphasis on high-quality proteins and essential fats. They are aimed at promoting muscle growth, optimizing hormonal health, and improving overall well-being. Within these pages, you have stumbled upon more than just recipes; you have unearthed a guide to a culinary experience that is both uncomplicated and enlightening.

As you embark on your carnivore journey, allow the principles and recipes in this cookbook to ignite your curiosity, encourage you to try new things, and fully embrace the incredible possibilities of a diet that has been around since the dawn of time. Keep in mind, the heart of this diet lies not in limitation, but in embracing the abundant nourishment that nature offers.

For those who are passionate about their health and vitality, this is just the beginning, not the end. May your dishes be filled with flavor, your well-being strong, and your enthusiasm unwavering. Here's to embracing a life enriched by the incredible benefits of the carnivore diet. Cheers to your well-being, vitality, and the exciting culinary journeys that lie ahead on this meat-centric path.

HAPPY

COOKING!